Xiomara Córdova
Araseli Jaimes

Gastric cancer and associated factors

Xiomara Córdova
Araseli Jaimes

Gastric cancer and associated factors

Gastric cancer in a Peruvian public hospital

ScienciaScripts

Imprint

Any brand names and product names mentioned in this book are subject to trademark, brand or patent protection and are trademarks or registered trademarks of their respective holders. The use of brand names, product names, common names, trade names, product descriptions etc. even without a particular marking in this work is in no way to be construed to mean that such names may be regarded as unrestricted in respect of trademark and brand protection legislation and could thus be used by anyone.

Cover image: www.ingimage.com

This book is a translation from the original published under ISBN 978-613-9-08304-6.

Publisher:
Sciencia Scripts
is a trademark of
Dodo Books Indian Ocean Ltd. and OmniScriptum S.R.L publishing group

120 High Road, East Finchley, London, N2 9ED, United Kingdom
Str. Armeneasca 28/1, office 1, Chisinau MD-2012, Republic of Moldova, Europe
Printed at: see last page
ISBN: 978-620-8-14501-9

DEDICATION

To God and our parents, for their valuable teachings, their unconditional love and for the support provided to achieve our goals.

INDEX

PREFACE

With more than 1.89 million new cases worldwide in 2020, gastric cancer represents one of the most common malignancies and is a public health concern in many countries. In terms of frequency, it ranks fifth and is the fourth leading cause of cancer-related death.

(1) Due to its late diagnosis, the 5-year survival rate is 20%. (2) According to the American Society Against Gastric Cancer in the United States, in the next few years about 27,510 cases of this cancer will be diagnosed and 10,730 people will die as a result, which represents 40.6% of those who die. (3)

(4) East Asia, Eastern Europe, South America and Central America are the areas most affected by this pathology. The Pan American Health Organization reports that more than 85,000 new cases of gastric carcinoma and 65,000 deaths are registered annually in the Americas. It is predicted that by 2030, Latin America and the Caribbean will experience a near doubling in the number of patients and deaths caused by this disease (3).

In Peru, according t o GLOBOCAN 2020 data, a total of 6300 (9%) incident cases of gastric cancer have been estimated, placing it in third place in frequency and first in mortality (14.2%). The most affected areas in this country are those in poor conditions in the highlands such as: Huancavelica, Ayacucho, Apurimac, Huanuco, Piura, Pasco, Cajamarca and Puno. The department with the highest incidence and mortality is Huánuco, with a mortality rate of 41.4/100,000 inhabitants (1).

There are multiple risk factors associated with this cancer, among the factors that increase the risk of this neoplasm are atrophic gastritis, intestinal metaplasia and dysplasia, obesity, low consumption of fruits and vegetables, among others. (5) According to Liming Shao and Peiwei Li, intestinal metaplasia is a risk factor for stomach cancer with an OR of 3.58. (6) On the other hand, Christine, Friedenreich and Ryder demonstrated a strong correlation between obesity and gastric tumor, affecting 80% of men and women. In this regard, the International Agency for Research on Cancer states that obesity is related to a greater probability of developing stomach cancer (7).

Finally, low consumption of fruits and vegetables increases the risk of gastric cancer, since these foods have protective, anti-inflammatory and anticarcinogenic properties. (8) In a systematic review, Poorolajal and Moradi demonstrated that the consumption of fruits and vegetables significantly reduced the risk of stomach cancer by 48% and 62%, respectively. (9) In a review in Chile, Montes V, et al. mention that the consumption of fruits and vegetables reduces the risk of developing this disease.(10)

Gastric carcinogenesis is a complex process, so identifying these factors and managing them could reduce the incidence of the disease. Therefore, endoscopic follow-up in patients is one of the solutions described for the control of premalignant lesions because it helps to identify cancer at an early stage, where it can be operated on and has a high probability of being cured.(11)

Regular physical activity is a useful measure for obesity because it has anti-inflammatory effects that reduce systemic levels of proinflammatory biomarkers.

by reducing adiposity (7) and with respect to the consumption of fruits and vegetables, it has been described that it reduces the risk of gastric cancer, thus having a protective role (8,12).

Due to its high frequency and mortality, stomach cancer in the department of Huánuco (Peru) should be considered an emerging public health problem. The literature describes many risk factors associated with gastric tumor, it is necessary to determine those that are most associated in our environment in order to generate promotion and prevention measures and provide early treatment to the patient.

CHAPTER I RESEARCH PROBLEM

Gastric cancer (GC) is a common pathology. It is estimated that in 2020 there were more than one million incident diagnoses and more than 600 thousand deaths due to this disease worldwide. Globally, it ranks fifth in frequency and fourth in mortality (1).

It has a wide geographical variation in incidence, regions such as Asia, Eastern Europe, Latin America have a higher incidence of GC; while Africa, North America and Northern Europe have a lower incidence. The importance of the study of GC lies in the development of adequate diagnostic, surgical and chemotherapy techniques, among others, to reduce mortality if an early diagnosis is made; since cases are currently recognized in advanced stages, when the prognosis is bleak and treatment is limited. (13,14)

Due to the high frequency of GC, it is considered a public health problem. Survival of all types of cancer overall is estimated at 68.9 % at five years, compared to gastric cancer, in which survival is only 32%.(15)

In Peru, according to 2020 predictions, GC is the third most common cancer; resulting in turn in the most lethal cancer for the Peruvian population. Geographic variation is also present in the interior of our country. Ruiz et al. demonstrated that the mortality rate for stomach cancer varies within Peru. Huánuco heads the list of departments with the highest incidence and mortality (41.4/100,000 inhabitants) for stomach cancer (16,17).

There are multiple risk factors associated with this neoplasm. Non-modifiable factors such as advanced age, male sex, ethnicity and genetic factors; and modifiable factors such as *Helicobacter pylori* infection (main factor), diet (low consumption of fruits and vegetables with low consumption of vitamins A and C), behavioral factors (tobacco and alcohol), as well as overweight/obesity and premalignant lesions. Additionally, the International Agency for Research on Cancer (IARC) includes other risk factors such as the rubber production industry, X-radiation and gamma radiation as carcinogenic agents with sufficient evidence in humans. (9,6,17)

CHAPTER II THEORETICAL FRAMEWORK

2.1 Background

International level

Shao et al. (China, 2018), conducted a systematic review entitled: "Gastric cancer risk among patients with gastric intestinal metaplasia". The objective was to assess the risk of GC among patients with intestinal metaplasia (IM). A total of 21 studies involving 402,636 participants and 4,535 patients with GC were included; all studies adopted histopathology for the diagnosis of IM. Statistically significant association was evidenced between IM and GC with a value of p<0.001, an OR of 3.58, 95% CI 2.71-4.73. Concluding that patients with IM were at higher risk of GC, especially incomplete IM (6).

Friedenreich and Ryder (Canada, 2020) conducted a systematic review of obesity in relation to GC, finding a strong association between obesity and GC with a RR= 4.8, affecting men and women in 80%.(7)

Lihu Gu and Yangfan Zhang (China, 2021) conducted a retrospective cohort study, which examined 607 patients with obesity-associated GC, the findings showed that overweight/obesity was a predictive factor (RR = 0.61, 95% CI: 0.37-0.99) with a p<0.0001 for GC prognosis.(18)

In a systematic review and meta-analysis by Poorolajal J et al (Iran, 2020), entitled: "Risk Factors for Stomach Cancer" aimed to provide information on nutritional and behavioral factors to address GC prevention programs. 232 studies were included in their review, of which 13 studies indicated that fruit consumption ($\geq$3 times/week) significantly decreased the risk of GC by 48%, with a value of p=0.001. On the other hand, 18 studies showed that consuming vegetables significantly reduced the risk of GC by 62% (p=0.001) (9).

Montes V, et al (2021) conducted a review in Chile on international strategies for the prevention of gastric cancer, where 28 studies were included. They mention that the consumption of fruits and vegetables reduces the risk of GC, the intake of more than 3 servings of fruits or vegetables per day reduces 0.48 and 0.62 times the risk of gastric tumor, respectively.(10)

Amiry et al. (Afghanistan, 2022), executed a case-control study. The aim of this research was to look for the association between Mediterranean diet and GC. A total of 270 individuals (90 cases and 180 controls) participated in the study. The assessment of dietary intake was performed by means of a food frequency questionnaire. From the evaluation of food itkthe results showed that GC patients presented a low intake of fruits (p≤0.001) and vegetables (p≤0.001). It was obtained that participants with a high DMS (mediterranean diet score) score were 83% less likely to present GC (19).

National level

Mendoza C. (2021). In his thesis on conditioning factors associated with the development of GC in hospitalized patients of the gastroenterology service of the Arzobispo Loayza National Hospital, his objective was to determine the conditioning factors associated with GC in the aforementioned hospital. The results showed a significant association between the following factors with GC: coming from the highlands or jungle, being overweight, having a Helicobacter pylori infection, having chronic atrophic gastritis and gastric polyps; with a value of p=<0.05. (20)

Castro M. (2020), in his research, identified chronic atrophic gastritis as one of the epidemiological clinical factors linked to stomach cancer, with an OR= 2.412, CI:95%, in patients at the Hospital Nacional Dos De Mayo (21).

Paucar E. (2019), in his study on risk factors associated with the development of GC, concludes that superficial chronic gastritis (p=0.0001), atrophic chronic gastritis (p=0.0005), metaplasia (p=0.0005), dysplasia (p=0.001), are risk factors for the development of GC.(22)

Quispe S. (2015), in her study on dietary patterns related to GC in patients treated at the Regional Institute of Neoplastic Diseases.
- Norte, found that a risk factor for the development of GC in these patients was insufficient consumption of dairy products, foods of animal origin, vegetables (OR=4.4), fruits (OR=30.0), with a p<0.001.(23)

Regional level

In Huanuco, 2016, Narciso and Eulogio, in their research study on Helicobacter pylori infection, socioeconomic level and dietary factors associated with GC, conducted in a public hospital, showed with respect to dietary factors significant relationship with gastric cancer and low intake of: garnish vegetables (cabbage, broccoli) with a p=0.000 (weekly), citrus fruits with a p=0.000 (weekly).(24)

In Huánuco, 2019, Rodríguez P. in his thesis mentions sociodemographic factors, harmful and dietary habits related to GC. In his conclusions, he established as "other epidemiological factors" related to gastric tumor the interval of fruit consumption in more than 10 days; the consumption of vegetables in an interval of more than 5 days.(25)

2.2. Gastric Cancer

Gastric cancer (GC) is a neoplasm located in the walls of the stomach. The Spanish Society of Oncology defines GC as any malignant tumor arising from the cells of any of the layers of the stomach. Most stomach cancers are adenocarcinomas, which are the most frequent histological type (> 90% of cases). Sarcomas, neuroendocrine tumors, gastrointestinal stromal tumors (GIST), lymphomas and other histologic categories have a lower incidence.

Epidemiology

GC ranks fifth in incidence (5.6%) of malignant tumors globally and fourth in cancer mortality (GLOBOCAN 2020). Its distribution presents important geographical, ethnic and socioeconomic differences.(4) Its geographical variety is one of its defining characteristics; in African countries, India and the United States, for example, the disease is rare. However, in countries such as China, Japan, Portugal, Colombia and Chile, among others, the mortality rate due to this pathology is significant.(5) Currently, 60% of gastric tumor cases in the world come from Korea, China and Japan. The areas most affected by GC are East Asia, Eastern Europe, Central and South America. According to the Pan American Health Organization (PAHO), more than 85,000 new cases of stomach cancer and 65,000 deaths from the disease are reported annually in the Americas. It is predicted that by 2030 the number of patients and deaths from GC will nearly double in Latin America and the Caribbean. (3)

In Peru it is the third most frequent neoplasm and the first in mortality (14.2%), the most affected areas of this country correspond to the poor highland regions (Huancavelica, Ayacucho, Apurímac, Cajamarca, Huánuco, Pasco, Piura and Puno). Huanuco is the department with the highest incidence and mortality (41.4/100,000 inhabitants) (1).

Etiopathogenesis

GC is multifactorial and involves a complex interaction of infectious agents (Helicobacter pylori and EpsteinBarr virus), environmental (high salt intake, tobacco use and diets poor in fiber, fruits and vegetables) and genetic factors (family history of GC) (11).

The development of neoplastic cells requires a change in the epithelium. The most important contributing factor is the bacterium H. pylori, which is contracted during childhood and can persist throughout life if not treated promptly. It has been identified as a carcinogen in 60-70% of cases. Its cytotoxic components, such as VacA toxin, CagA and NapA protein, cause it to infiltrate the stomach mucosa. Likewise, the risk of developing GC due to infection by this bacterium is 2 to 20 times (13,26).

Between 40% to 30% of gastric cancers are caused by deficient consumption of fruits and vegetables. In 18% of cases, smoking and in 13%, Epstein Barr virus infections. This malignant neoplasm is 3 to 18 times more likely in the presence of atrophic gastritis(13).

Pathophysiology

Gastric cancer is related to H. pylori infection, which if left untreated can persist throughout life and provoke a chronic inflammatory response that can cause a series of events leading to neoplasia. The preneoplastic cascade consists of the following stages: atrophic gastritis, intestinal metaplasia, dysplasia and finally gastric carcinoma.(11,13)

Neoplasia is associated with oxidative stress caused by nitric oxide synthase produced by inflammatory cells in response to infection. Moreover, latoxin VacA from the bacterium causes epithelial cell death and allows entry of carcinogens and invasion of the neoplasm; the toxin CagA modifies the shape of epithelial cells and release IL-8, which triggers an inflammatory response.(13)

Ranking

The degree of penetration of gastric carcinoma into the wall determines whether it is early (affecting the mucosa and submucosa) or advanced (invades the other layers of the gastric wall). Taking into account the location, the entire stomach is vulnerable to cancer... "the predominance existing in the distal third four decades ago has been decreasing in favor of an absolute and relative increase in the upper third, mainly in the cardial region". (13)

The most commonly used categorization system for stomach tumors is Lauren's classification which, based on tumor histology, describes two main types of gastric adenocarcinomas: diffuse and intestinal. The intestinal type represents up to 70% of cases (27) and is characterized by the adoption of the cells to a form more similar to the gastric gland, has a better prognosis compared to the diffuse form, which is characterized by being undifferentiated, invasive and presenting a family history.(28)

On the other hand, the classification system of Nakamura and Sugano based on the carcinomatous cells observed around the mucosa, divides it into undifferentiated and differentiated carcinoma. (5) Finally, GC is divided into four groups according to the 2010 World Health Organization (WHO) classification:

- Epithelial.
- Non-epithelial.
- Malignant lymphomas.
- Secondary tumors.

In turn, four major histological types are recognized in the epithelial group:

- The tubular.
- Papillary.
- The mucinous.
- Poorly cohesive (includes signet ring cell carcinoma), plus rare histological variants (29).

The Borrmann classification, based on the morphological characteristics of gastric tumors, divides them into five types depending on the macroscopic appearance:

➤ Type I: represents polypoid or fungal cancers.

➤ Type II: includes ulcerative lesions surrounded by raised borders.

➤ Type III: represents ulcerated lesions that infiltrate the gastric wall.

- ➤ Type IV: includes diffusely infiltrating tumors.

- ➤ Type V: gastric cancers are unclassifiable cancers (26).

Clinical picture

The clinical presentation of GC depends on the stage of the disease at the time of diagnosis. In the early stage it is usually asymptomatic, so early detection is usually not possible. (5) Therefore, due to the vague and nonspecific symptoms that characterize it, many patients are diagnosed with advanced stage disease. (26)

Abdominal pain (62% to 91%) and weight loss (22% to 61%) are the most frequently reported symptoms. In addition to other symptoms such as anorexia (5% to 40%), nausea and vomiting (6% to 40%), as a result of obstruction due to tumor growth or loss of gastric distension. In proximal lesions (cardioesophageal junction) dysphagia predominates, but in distal lesions (antrum and pylorus), early gastric fullness. (26,28)

Weight loss should not be underestimated. Dewys et al. found that >80% of 179 patients with advanced gastric cancer had experienced >10% weight loss before diagnosis. Furthermore, the survival time of patients who lost weight was substantially shorter than that of patients who did not.(26,28)

Diagnosis

Gastroscopy (upper endoscopy) with biopsy is the standard diagnostic method for GC. (30) Upper endoscopy is the most precise, descriptive and practical study to diagnose this pathology, it allows us to obtain biopsies and perform palliative and therapeutic procedures in early and limited lesions. It is important to take multiple biopsies during endoscopy since more than 7 samples have up to 98% sensitivity for diagnosis. Plastic lymphitis (diffuse histological type of GC) is difficult to diagnose by endoscopy (28).

Barium contrasted imaging studies are useful to diagnose proximal or distal lesions. Three-phase computed tomography (CT) is indicated to evaluate resectability and staging (sensitivity 50 - 70%). Besides being the best study to find metastases. Endoscopic ultrasound is useful in patients who are candidates for wide mucosal or submucosal resection (28).

Treatment

This disease is mainly treated by surgical procedures. Resectability, tumor location in the stomach, histologic type, extent of resection, surgical margin, type of reconstruction and palliative surgery are the objectives evaluated i n surgical c a n d i d a t e s . For surgical treatment, GC has been divided into early and locally advanced resectable (28).

The tumor and surrounding affected tissues should be resected along with lymphatic resection. Subtotal gastrectomy is associated with improved nutritional status and better quality of life (5).

Forecast

Studies show a five-year survival rate of 30.4%, all depending on proper and timely diagnosis and staging. Early stage and correct diagnosis contribute to 66.9% survival, while late stage contributes to 5%. As it is an aggressive disease, it is crucial to monitor the patient and provide adequate intensive treatment (13).

2.3. Premalignant lesions

Gastric premalignant conditions include *Helicobacter pylori* infection, gastric atrophy, intestinal metaplasia and dysplasia. The etiologic role of H. pylori is undisputed. (31) Atrophic gastritis, intestinal metaplasia and dysplasia are considered high-risk lesions for gastric cancer because of the damage they cause to the stomach during the disease process. (5)

The presence of precancerous lesions and their identification can also take time.

several years. Therefore, endoscopic follow-up in high-risk patients can help to identify malignant lesions at an early stage when they are still operable and have a high probability of being cured. (11)

The diagnosis of premalignant lesions requires histology. The Sydney protocol is recommended. Biopsies should be sent separately in two flasks (antrum-angle and body) (31).

In a Swedish study of a large population of 405,000 people with endoscopy showing normal or altered mucosa, it was shown that after 20 years of follow-up one in 256 patients with normal mucosa developed gastric cancer, while this risk was one in 85 cases with atrophic gastritis, one in 39 cases with intestinal metaplasia, and one in 19 cases with dysplasia. Therefore, the European Society of Pathology recommends that patients with extensive intestinal atrophy or metaplasia should have an endoscopic follow-up every 3 years (32).

A 10-year follow-up study reported that the rates of progression to GC for patients with atrophic gastritis, intestinal metaplasia, mild dysplasia and severe dysplasia were 0.8%, 1.8%, 4% and 33%, respectively.

GASTRIC ATROPHY

The National Cancer Institute defines it as a condition characterized by thinning of the inner lining of the gastric wall and loss of glandular cells in that lining which emit substances that help with digestion. It may be caused by H. pylori i n f e c t i o n or by other autoimmune conditions. Gastric atrophy may increase the risk of stomach cancer.

Atrophy of the oxyntic area is a major risk condition for GC, and both H. pylori infection and autoimmune gastritis are the events that produce this oxyntic atrophy. Autoimmune gastritis of the gastric fundus is the one associated with pernicious anemia. It has been described that the prevalence of GC in this disease is 1-3% and these patients are 2-3 times more at risk of developing this neoplasm (11,32).

Epidemiology

GC develops over a long period of years to decades, therefore the frequency of gastric atrophy is very low before the age of 40 years (<5%) and the percentage of GC patients younger than 40 years corresponds to 5.9%. A study carried out in an area with a high incidence of GC reported a prevalence of 57 % of chronic atrophic degastritis (11).

Gastric mucosal atrophy and intestinal metaplasia confer a high risk for the development of GC, as they constitute the context in which intestinal-type gastric dysplasia and gastric adenocarcinoma develop (33).

Ranking

The risk of GC is classified according to the OLGA (Operative Link of Gastritis Assessment) system based on the degree of atrophy and its location (11,31).

Diagnosis

Gastric atrophy is rare before the age of 40 years. In the absence of focal lesions or family history, the search for premalignant lesions could be focused on those over 40 years of age. Endoscopy has poor diagnostic performance in the West, so the diagnosis of gastric atrophy, intestinal metaplasia requires systematic biopsies of the body and antrum. First-degree relatives of GC patients have 2 to 10 times higher risk of GC and higher frequency and earliness of GA. The modified Sydney protocol includes 5 biopsies (2 in the antrum and body and one in the angle) and is the most widely accepted (5).

INTESTINAL METAPLASIA

Intestinal metaplasia (IM) is a premalignant lesion characterized by loss of the gastric epithelium and appearance of glands with intestinal phenotype, which replace the original ones and their secretions. It is due to the presence of H. pylori infection, smoking and high salt consumption mainly (5,13).

Epidemiology

The overall prevalence is 7% and affects men and women equally, increasing with age. In a study conducted in an area with a high incidence of GC, a prevalence of IM of 38% was reported. The overall progression to gastric cancer ranges from 1.8-6.4% and this varies in different scenarios: progression of type III MI up to 10%, progression with dysplasia up to 79% and the prevalence of cancer in MI is 11% (5,11). (5,11).

Ranking

According to the histological classification of Jass and Filipe, gastric IM is divided into complete (type I or small bowel) and incomplete (type IIA/II or enterocolic and type IIB/III or colonic). IM can also be classified by its extension into focal (one affected area) and diffuse (2 or more affected areas) which is determined during upper endoscopy (5).

Incomplete IM and diffuse involvement are associated with an increased risk of neoplastic progression. In a recent study in Spain, gastric carcinoma developed in 18.2% of 88 patients with incomplete intestinal metaplasia, while it occurred in only one (0.96%) of 104 patients with complete intestinal metaplasia after a follow-up of 12.8 years (5,33).

It is suggested that the risk of GC be staged according to the OLGIM system for IM, which should be included in the histologic report. A Chinese study suggests that body-predominant gastritis and OLGIM II-IV are significantly associated with GC risk(31).

Diagnosis

According to the latest European consensus for the diagnosis of gastric atrophy and metaplasia, at l e a s t 4 biopsies of the proximal and distal stomach should be taken (2 of greater curvature and 2 of lesser curvature). In cases of already diagnosed gastric IM, if there is a family history or the patient is of a high-risk race for gastric cancer, the American Society for Gastrointestinal Endoscopy (ASGE) suggests performing endoscopic follow-up and continuing it at established intervals according to individual risk (5).

DYSPLASIA

Dysplasia is described as cellularity with a neoplastic phenotype confined to glandular structures (13).

Epidemiology

A previous study by Pelayo Correa conducted in an area with a high incidence of GC reported a prevalence of dysplasia of 10% in individuals over 40 years of age (1). The annual progression from dysplasia to GC varies between 0% and 73% in one year, partly due to diagnostic variability (31).

In the Netherlands, a cohort study showed an annual incidence of 0.1% for gastric atrophy, 0.25% for IM, 0.6% for mild to moderate dysplasia, and 6% for severe dysplasia (31).

Ranking

Dysplasia is divided into two categories, based on dysplastic alterations according to their gradation, in low and high grade. The purpose of this is to try to evaluate the risk and guide the therapeutic attitude (34).

Other classifications of importance correspond to the modified Vienna

Classification and the WHO classification.

➢ Vienna classification. It classifies it in 5 categories: negative for neoplasia, undefined for neoplasia, low grade neoplasia, high grade neoplasia and invasion of the submucosa (35).

➢ WHO classification for dysplasia: negative for dysplasia, undefined paradysplasia, low grade dysplasia, high grade dysplasia and cancer (31).

Diagnosis

Dysplasia can be found anywhere in the stomach, but most often it is found in the antrum. Also most of the time dysplasia is discovered incidentally during screening endoscopies. (11) Regarding its management, high grade lesions require endoscopic resection, due to their potential for progression to carcinoma and coexistence with carcinoma. (11)

2.4. Overweight/Obesity

The term obesity refers to an excess of fat in the body, being a chronic metabolic disease, resulting from a positive energy balance where energy intake exceeds energy expenditure. Obesity is evaluated by anthropometry (ratio between weight and height) and waist circumference, which gives us an estimate of body fat. According to the WHO, obesity is a chronic disease, a product of poor lifestyle choices, recognized as a disease of body weight regulation. (36- 40) Overweight/obesity is strongly related to stomach cancer, according to Yang's review, which concludes that the higher the body mass index, the higher the risk of GC in non-Asians. (41)

Recently, they have defined obesity as a systemic, multi-organ, metabolic and chronic inflammatory disease, determined by the interrelation between genomic and environmental factors, which corresponds to an alteration in the function of adipose tissue, both quantitatively and qualitatively, in its capacity to store fat, which leads to lipoinflammation (42).

Risk factors include endocrinological pathologies such as hypothyroidism, Cushing's syndrome, hypogonadism and hypothalamic lesions associated with hyperphagia, as well as socioeconomic, demographic, physical activity, lifestyle and behavioral factors (36).

In lifestyle we have: the dietary factor, where a higher intake of foods rich in fat, salt, sugars and specific products such as chips, processed meats, red meat, sweets, implies a disproportion in energy intake, predisposing the subject to obesity (36-37).

Likewise, decreased physical activity, sedentary behaviors, increased use of automation of work activities, modern methods of transportation and increased urban living have been associated with an increased risk of obesity (37).

Ranking

Adipose tissue is distributed in the body through a visceral store and a subcutaneous store. Accordingly, the classification given by the WHO and a panel of experts from the National Institute of Health (NIH) is based on the BMI, which corresponds to the ratio between weight in kilograms and the square of height in meters (36).

Taking into account the Deurenberg equation for estimating body fat, shown by the following formula: % body fat = 1.2 (BMI) + 0.23 (age) - 10.8 (sex) - 5.4. Where, sex = 1 for males, and 0 for females. The ranking is given as follows:

o   Low Weight: <18.5 kg/m^2
o   Normal weight: 18.5-24.9 kg/ m^2
o   Overweight: 25-29.9 kg/ m^2
o   Obesity grade 1: 30-34.9 kg/ m^2
o   Obesity grade 2: 35 to 39,9 kg/ m^2
o   Grade 3 obesity: $\geq$ 40 kg/ m^2 . (36)

In a review by Yang, another classification for overweight/obesity was used, where the Asia-Pacific classification of overweight (23.0 $\leq$ BMI < 24.9) and obesity (BMI $\geq$ 25.0) (42).

We can also observe the creation of additional subcategories such as that of theSEEDO in 2007 where it subdivides overweight into grade 1 (25- 26.9 kg/ m^2) and grade 2 (27-29.9 kg/ m^2), we also see a change in the nomenclature for grade 3 obesity, also called morbid, extending it to 49.9 kg/ m^2 and the category of extreme obesity (super morbid) with a value equal to or greater than 50 kg/ m^2 . (42). Therefore, the calculation of BMI greater than or equal to 30 kg/m^2 is considered obesity (36).

Pathophysiology

The adipocyte is the functional unit of adipose tissue, its main function is to store excess energy in the form of triglycerides and to be released when there is a need for energy; it also plays a role in the energy balance, due to its bioactive factors called adipokines, which include leptin and adiponectin giving a dysregulation of the secretory profile of adipose tissue and adipocyte, with an alteration in an increase in the serum level of the former and a decrease in adiponectin. An obese person has a higher lean mass accompanied by a higher basal metabolic rate, cardiac output and blood pressure. (43,44)

The cellular microenvironment is made up of M1 macrophages, T cells, fibroblasts, and adipocytes, thus having an inflammatory secretory profile, increasing their number due to the infiltration of monocytes (43).

The adipocyte develops by two processes: by hypertrophy that reaches a critical size threshold and by hyperplasia when this limit is exceeded, the hypertrophied adipocyte presents a dysfunction in its activity due to a decrease in insulin sensitivity, increasing intracellular stress, leading to an increase in inflammatory factors. The interaction of hypertrophic adipocytes with macrophages generates insufficient angiogenic capacity, favoring the development of chronic hypoxia, apoptosis and a greater release of proinflammatory cytokines (43,45).

Hypertrophy leads to an alteration of the leptin secretory profile, insulin insensitivity, increasing endoplasmic reticulum stress, resulting in basal lipolysis (overflow hypothesis) (43).

In adults, the gain of adipose tissue is mostly due to hypertrophy, where a transitional inflammatory state occurs, with the number of adipocytes remaining stable. As inflammation is perpetuated, metabolic behavior is modified, becoming systemic through circulation (43).

Visceral adipose tissue becomes the first store of triglycerides in the face of the incompetence of subcutaneous adipose tissue, the increase of fat deposition at the central level is considered a risk factor (43). The increase in intra-abdominal pressure observed in these individuals increases the risk of gastric reflux, Barrett's esophagus and esophageal adenocarcinoma (44).

Obese women have a greater disposition to store fat at the subcutaneous tissue level, in the gluteal-femoral region, while men tend to have more centralized visceral fat, which is more active in the production of leptin and adiponectin (37,42).

Brown adipose tissue (BAT), which dissipates energy as heat and therefore performs adaptive thermogenesis, is also strongly innervated and vascularized, attributing to it the anti-obesity property. (42) the International Agency for Research on Cancer (IARC) established that excess body fat is associated with an increased risk of at least 13 different types of cancer, including stomach cancer, it is believed that regular physical activity has anti-inflammatory effects by reducing systemic levels of pro-inflammatory biomarkers and increases the levels of anti-inflammatory biomarkers at least by decreasing adiposity. (9)

2.5.   Dietary habits

Fruits and vegetables are edible parts of plants, whether grown or harvested, in raw or minimally processed form (washed, trimmed and peeled). It has its exclusions such as: starchy tubers, legumes and cereals, nuts, medicinal plants and ultra-processed products. fruits and vegetables are an important source of nutrients, fiber, water, phytochemicals and antioxidants. (45-47)

It has been described that a higher consumption of fruits and vegetables leads to a lower risk of GC, thus having a protective role, whose associations have been found in greater quantity among greenish-yellow vegetables due to their carotenoid and isothiocyanate properties; and among fruits we have citrus fruits for their content in flavanones and vitamin C, while their low consumption is associated with a higher risk of developing GC. (49-51)

Ranking

The WHO and FAO currently recommend a minimum consumption of 400 g of fruits and vegetables each day, i.e. five portions of 80 g each. However, the optimal amount depends on various factors such as age, sex and physical activity. Eating 7-8 servings per day is associated with a lower risk of disease, so it is advisable to consume 2.5 servings of vegetables and 2 servings of fruits per day for a 2000 calorie diet. (46,47)

The classification of fruits and vegetables according to their color: dark green vegetables: broccoli, spinach, romaine, kale and turnip; red and orange vegetables: tomatoes, red peppers, carrots and pumpkin and in other vegetables: lettuce, green beans, onions, cucumbers, cabbage, celery, zucchini, mushrooms and green peppers. Fruits include fresh fruits such as oranges, apples, bananas, grapes, melons, berries and raisins (46).

The recommended amounts range from 2 to 3 whole fruits per day, taking as an estimate that one cup is equivalent to the size of a fist of the hand and this to a medium sized fruit. I n   vegetables we have that the volume should be half of the daily intake, that is, 2 to 3 cups per day, with an equivalence of half a cup (4 ounces) of a rounded fist of cooked vegetables.(46)

In Europe, the average consumption of vegetables and legumes is 220 g per day and of fruit 166 g per day, giving an average consumption between fruit and vegetables of 386 g per day.(47) Food frequency questionnaires (FFQ) are widely used dietary surveys that provide significant information on intake over a long period of time.(52)

Two patterns are identified in the FFQ: personal interviews and self-administered FFQs. In a case control study, it was seen that most FFQs included fruits, such as apples, pears, oranges, bananas, grapes, peaches, berries, watermelon; and vegetables such as cauliflower, broccoli, carrots, lettuce, cabbage, tomato, green bell pepper, cucumber and onion, were the most common. The frequency of consumption of each food group per servings per day was obtained by summing the consumption frequencies and then classifying them into tertiles.(50)

Another study identified two common dietary patterns: the first, I call 'prudent/healthy', (fruits and vegetables, fish) labeled as 'rich in vitamins, vegetables and fruits, the second pattern was 'unhealthy', with high loads of meat, bread, high-fat dairy products and sweets.(52)

In another study where the FFQ was applied, it was seen that for subjects who were in the habit of consuming fruits, they were asked to report their frequency and quantity of consumption. The frequency category ranged from "never or less than 1 per month" to "6-7 per week". These food frequencies and their amounts were converted to consumption in grams per day, using household units. The median daily consumption w a s   179 g of vegetables and 157 g of fruits. The most frequently consumed vegetables in this population were green beans, cauliflower and lettuce and of the fruits consumed were apples, pears and oranges (54).

Pathophysiology

Fruits and vegetables have a high antioxidant power, such as polyphenols (flavonoids, flavonols, flavones, isoflavones and anthocyanins) that provide the organism with a protective factor against GC. Citrus fruits among their properties contain: vitamin C, carotenoids, flavanones such as hesperitin, which act by inhibiting the proliferation and migration of GC cells. The fiber in fruits and vegetables act as nitrate scavengers, preventing the formation of carcinogenic nitrous compounds.(45,49)

Fiber is in soluble form as pectin and in insoluble form as cellulose and hemicellulose, among the phytochemicals we find vitamin A, C, E, thiamine. Fruits and vegetables also contain minerals such as magnesium, zinc and potassium; they also contain carbohydrates in the form of fructose and starches. (48)

Oxidative stress produces free radicals and peroxide, which are produced by radiation or environmental pollutants that become toxic in our organism, characterized by a high reactivity, which is responsible for their cytotoxic and genotoxic effects. Their excess causes hyperactivation of phosphorylation and oxidation of proteins, generating a chronic inflammatory state, uncontrolled proliferation and cellular degeneration (45,54).

Fruits and vegetables as antioxidants, according to their composition it is observed that in 200 g of fruits there are 500 mg of total polyphenols. This property depends on the hydroxylation power, position and substitution of its hydroxyl groups, its structure can be simple or complex, ascorbic acid is one of the best natural antioxidants. polyphenol detoxifies ROS and free radicals, acts as an anti-inflammatory by inhibiting cyclooxygenase, lipoxygenase and nitric oxide synthase. RNS in the presence of acid pH form nitrating/nitrosating species that favor the formation of carcinogenic nitrosamines leading to GC (45).

The consumption of fruit juices has a high percentage of polyphenols that increase the antioxidant capacity in plasma. Thus, purple/blue, red and green fruits help t o reduce the risk of cancer (48).

Polyphenol metabolism begins with the hydrolyzation of flavonoids to aglycones, which can be absorbed in smaller quantities by the buccal epithelium; they then pass to the gastrointestinal tract, being reduced to monomers, and finally pass into circulation, reaching the liver to be transformed into active metabolites (46).

Flavonoids and their metabolites are bioactive molecules with the ability to interact with intracellular signaling pathways; thus having an antitumor function. It has been described that the effects of polyphenols at the level of the gastrointestinal tract have a greater antioxidant capacity, before being metabolized and absorbed into the bloodstream(46).

The consumption of vegetables brings many benefits to the organism, as they have sulfur compounds, with protective effects, vitamins, carotenoids and phytochemicals with anti-inflammatory and antioxidant activity, which transmit anticarcinogenic effects. Therefore, consuming little or no fruit increases the risk of CG (50).

CHAPTER III METHODOLOGY

Scope

The study was carried out in the city of Huánuco, province of Huánuco, belonging to the region of the same name. It was carried out at hospital II EsSalud, in the gastroenterology service.

Population

1. **P. Target:** The total population of patients seen in the gastroenterology service of hospital II EsSalud, who attended for gastric digestive pathology during the study period 2022.

2. **P. Accessible:** The total population of patients seen in the gastroenterology service of hospital II EsSalud who attended for gastric digestive pathology during the time of study 2022.

3. **P. Eligible:** Patients who meet the selection criteria.

Inclusion criteria

- Patients undergoing endoscopy in the gastroenterology service of hospital II EsSalud Huánuco.
- Patients with anatomopathologic report for gastric pathology of the gastroenterology service of hospital II EsSalud Huánuco.
- Patients diagnosed with gastric cancer by histology.
- Patients with complete medical histories in more than 80% with respect to the variables under study.
- Patients who agree to participate and sign or accept the informed consent clauses.

Exclusion criteria

- Patients from a service other than gastroenterology who do not require a diagnosis of gastric cancer.
- Patients who do not wish to participate or decide to withdraw.
- Patients who do not complete the questionnaire.

- Patients with incomplete medical records.

Unit of analysis:

A patient with gastric pathology who attended the gastroenterology service with endoscopic procedure and anatomopathological report.

Sample

The sample size consisted of 245 patients with an anatomopathologic report. It was found using the Epidat 3.1 program, with a proportion o f 46.2%, 95% confidence level. The sample was taken through systematic probability sampling.

Type of study

The level of research is observational.

Research design

The design used for this research was: observational, analytical, retrospective and cross-sectional.

- **It is observational:** Because it only merited observing the behavior of the variable under study without manipulation.
- **It is analytical:** Because it was necessary to analyze the factors that are associated with gastric cancer and those that are not associated by means of statistical techniques. It is correlational.
- **It is retrospective:** because the data collected were from the past 2022 and were obtained from the hospital's medical records.
- **It is transversal:** Because only one measurement was made.

Methods, techniques and instruments

The respective coordination was carried out according to the protocol, requesting the competent authorities of the Hospital II EsSalud - Huánuco, to execute the research process. Once authorization was obtained, the selected patients were informed of the reasons for the study by means of informed consent on the same day of the survey, and the corresponding information was subsequently collected.

A questionnaire of questions applied as a survey to the subjects of the selected sample was used, which was subjected to a validation process by the experts; a data c o l l e c t i o n form was also used, which had as a secondary source the clinical history of the patients under study.

Validation and reliability of the instrument

The data collection instrument was validated by 4 experts, who independently evaluated the clarity, objectivity, updating, organization, sufficiency, intentionality, consistency, coherence, methodology and relevance of the questions in the questionnaire. They obtained an average score of 90.75.

Reliability was evaluated with a pilot test, obtaining a Cronbach's Alpha of 0.76, which indicates that the instrument used in the research was reliable.

Procedure

Data collection was carried out by the principal investigators and two surveyors, all trained in the format of the data collection form and the questionnaire.

Tabulation and data analysis

Once the information was collected, the data were grouped, ordered and classified in a digital format in Excel and then imported into the SPSS Statistical Software (version 21) for the elaboration and representation of the respective frequency tables and graphs for each variable according to its dimensions. The Chi-Square statistical test (X^2) was used to look for the association between two qualitative variables within the same population. The level of statistical significance used was 5% ($p < 0.05$), with a confidence interval of 95%, which reflects statistical significance.

Ethical considerations

The principles established in the Declaration of Helsinki, Belmont Report, CIOMS guidelines, Declaration on Bioethics and Human Rights, UNESCO, Nuremberg Code were taken into account.
This study was approved by the ethics committee of the EAP of human medicine of the UNHEVAL and approved by the Hospital II EsSalud Huánuco.

A total of 245 questionnaires were applied to patients in the gastroenterology service of hospital II EsSalud, of which 145 (59.2%) were female and 100 (40.8%) were male; the distribution was skewed towards the female sex. The mean age of the participants was 58.8 years, with a minimum of 26 and a maximum of 90 years.

Table 1. Demographic characteristics of patients with gastric cancer in the gastroenterology service of hospital II EsSalud 2022 (n=245).

Feature	Frequency	Percentage
Genre		
Female	145	59.2%
Male	100	40.8%
Marital status		
Single	57	23.3%
Married	114	46.5%
Cohabitant	26	10.6%
Separated	17	6.9%
Widower	31	12.7%
Occupation		
Dependent work	76	31.0%
Self-employment	51	20.8%
Farmer	5	2.0%
Housewife	85	34.7%
Others	28	11.4%
Family history		
yes	18	7.3%
no	225	91.8%
Relationship		
Parents	6	33.3%
Brothers	5	27.7%
Grandparents	1	5.6%
Uncles	4	22.2%
Nephews	2	11.2%
Socioeconomic level		
NSE A	1	0.4%
NSE B	0	0.0%
NSE C	11	4.5%
NSE D	91	37.1%
NSE E	142	58.0%
Helicobacter Pylori		
Positive	186	75.9%
Negative	59	24.1%
Age		
Under 76 years old	225	91.8%
over 76 years old	20	8.2%

frequency were those under 76 years of age, 225 (91.8%). In terms of marital status, 114 (46.5%) were found to be married, being the most common. With respect to occupation, the most frequent job was that of housewife with a total of 85 (34.7%), followed by dependent work with a total of 76 (31%).

Those with a family history of gastric cancer were 18 (7.3%) of the participants and the predominant one was parental kinship 6 (2.4%). In the socioeconomic level (SES), the most frequent results were those of SES E with a total of 142 (58%). Patients diagnosed with positive Helicobacter pylori were 186 (%75.9). (Table 1).

Regarding the clinical characteristics of the 245 patients of the gastroenterology service, a total of 24 (9.8%) patients with gastric cancer and 221 (90.2%) without gastric cancer were obtained. Diffuse adenocarcinoma was the most frequent 12 (50.0%). R e g a r d i n g intestinal metaplasia it was found that 166 (67.7%) patients had it, being complete metaplasia the one with the highest histological frequency 83 (50.0%).

There were 130 (53.1%) patients with overweight and 21 (8.6%) with obesity. There was a predominance of low fruit consumption 138 (56.3%) and 105 (42.9%) participants had a low consumption of vegetables (Table 2).

Tabla 2. Características clínicas de los pacientes con cáncer gástrico del servicio de gastroenterología del hospital II EsSalud 2022 (n=245)		
Característica	Frecuencia	Porcentaje
Cáncer gástrico		
Si	24	9.8%
No	221	90.2%
Histología de cáncer gástrico		
Adenocarcinoma intestinal	8	33.3%
Adenocarcinoma difuso	12	50.0%
Otro	4	16.7%
Atrofia Gástrica		
Si	19	7.8%
No	226	92.2%
Metaplasia		
si	166	67.7%
no	79	32.3%
Histología de metaplasia		
Metaplasia completa	83	50.0%
Metaplasia incompleta	45	27.1%
Mixto	38	22.9%
Displasia		
Si	6	2.5%
No	239	97.5%
Sobrepeso		
Si tiene	130	53.1%
No tiene	115	46.9%
Obesidad		
Si tiene	21	8.6%
No tiene	224	91.4%
consumo de frutas		
Alto consumo	107	43.7%
Bajo consumo	138	56.3%
consumo de verduras		
Alto consumo	140	57.1%
Bajo consumo	105	42.9%

With respect to the association of the variables, an analysis was performed, obtaining PR (prevalence ratio) as a measure of association. A statistically significant association was observed between gastric cancer and fruit consumption (X^2 =4.6599, p=0.0309), PR: 1.47 (CI:95%,1.15-1.86), resulting in the low fruit consumption ($\leq$7 servings/week) as a risk factor. Likewise, a significant association was found with low vegetable consumption (X^2 =7.2838, p=0.0070), PR: 1.77 (CI:95%,1.31-2.40). On the other hand, a significant association was also

found with the age group older than 76 years with a value of X2= 3.9777, p= 0.0461; PR: 3.06 (CI:95%,1.22-7.70); with gender (X2=11.3493, p=0.0008), PR: 2.02 (CI:95%,1.51-2.69), resulting in the sex
male as a risk factor and with family history of gastric cancer (X^2 =5.0823, p= 0.0242), PR: 3.54 (CI:95%,1.38-9.07).

No significant association was found with the following study variables: gastric atrophy (X^2 =0.4789, p=0.4889), intestinal metaplasia
with family history of gastric cancer (X^2 =5.0823, p= 0.0242), PR: 3.54 (CI:95%,1.38-9.07).
No significant association was found with the following study variables: gastric atrophy (X2=0.4789, p=0.4889), intestinal metaplasia (X2=2.2486, p=0.1337), dysplasia (X2=1.609, p=0.2046), overweight (X2=0.0131, p=0.9090), obesity (X2=2.2249, p=0.1358) and Helicobacter pylori infection (see Table 3).

Tabla 3. Análisis bivariado de factores asociados a cáncer gástrico en pacientes del hospital II EsSalud, Huánuco 2022 (n=245)

Características	CÁNCER GÁSTRICO				x^2	p	RP	IC 95		
	Si tiene		No tiene							
	n	%	n	%				Inf	;	Sup
Lesiones premalignas										
Atrofia Gástrica										
Presente	1	5.3%	18	94.7%	0.4789	0.4889*	0.51	0.07	;	3.66
Ausente	23	10.2%	203	89.8%						
Metaplasia intestinal										
Presente	13	7.8%	153	92.2%	2.2486	0.1337*	0.78	0.53	;	1.14
Ausente	11	13.9%	68	86.1%						
Displasia										
Presente	2	33.3%	4	66.7%	1.609	0.2046**	4.6	0.88	;	23.83
Ausente	22	9.2%	217	90.8%						
Sobrepeso										
Si tiene	13	10.0%	117	90.0%	0.0131	0.9090*	1.02	0.69	;	1.50
No tiene	11	9.6%	104	90.4%						
Obesidad										
Si tiene	4	19.1%	17	80.9%	2.2249	0.1358*	2.16	0.79	;	5.91
No tiene	20	8.9%	204	91.1%						
Consumo de frutas										
Bajo consumo	19	13.8%	119	86.2%	4.6599	0.0309**	1.47	1.15	;	1.86
Alto consumo	5	4.7%	102	95.3%						
Consumo de verduras										
Bajo consumo	17	16.2%	88	83.8%	7.2838	0.0070**	1.77	1.31	;	2.40
Alto consumo	7	5.0%	133	95.0%						
Edad										
Mayor 76 años	5	25.0%	15	75.0%	3.9777	0.0461**	3.06	1.22	;	7.70
Menor igual 76 años	19	8.4%	206	91.6%						
Género										
Masculino	18	18.0%	82	82.0%	11.3493	0.0008**	2.02	1.51	;	2.69
Femenino	6	4.1%	139	95.9%						
Infección por HP										
Positivo	15	8.1%	171	91.9%	2.6203	0.1055*	0.81	0.58	;	1.11
Negativo	9	15.3%	50	84.7%						
Antecedente familiar										
Si	5	27.8%	13	72.2%	5.0823	0.0242**	3.54	1.38	;	9.07
No	19	8.4%	208	91.6%						
Nivel socioeconómico										
NSE bajo	19	13.4%	123	86.6%	3.9935	0.0457**	1.42	1.12	;	1.8
NSE alto	5	4.9%	98	95.1%						

*Chi cuadrado

**Corrección de Yates

HP: Helicobacter pylori

NSE: Nivel socioeconómico

CHAPTER V DISCUSSION

Gastric cancer is one of the most frequent neoplasms in the world. Incidence varies between geographic regions, and is higher in East Asian countries, Europe and some areas of Latin America, with the highest mortality rates mainly in Japan, Korea and China. (56-57) In Peru, the cancers with the highest mortality rates were those of the prostate, stomach, liver, among others. Huanuco is the department that tops the list at the national level for having gastric cancer and the highest mortality rate for this tumor (58).

In our investigation premalignant lesions, such as gastric atrophy (p=0.4889), intestinal metaplasia (p=0.1337) and dysplasia (p=0.2046) did not have a statistically significant association with the presence of gastric cancer diagnosed by pathological anatomy. In this regard, Akbari M., et al. and Spence A, et al. in their investigations point out that the incidence of GC in patients with GA and IM is low (59-60). Ortiz J et al., in their study point out that 46.2% of patients with gastric cancer presented these premalignant lesions. (61) On the other hand, Jonathan WJ and Feng Z (62); Antonio T, Cortés P, et al.
(63) described premalignant lesions as risk factors for gastric tumor. Shao L, et al. evidenced significant association between IM and GC (p<0.001), with an OR of 3.58, 95% CI 2.71-4.73. (6)

In our study it was determined that there is no statistically significant association of overweight/obesity (p=0.9090/ p=0.1358) with gastric cancer. The results found in our study coincide with Paucar; (64) Vallejo and Orellana; who point out that overweight/obesity is not a risk factor.
(65) A meta-analysis developed in Iran showed that overweight/obesity had no significant effect on GC (p=0.240) with an OR: 0.89 (95 % CI 0.74-1.08) (9). Jun X, et al. in their meta-analysis describes obesity as a risk factor with an OR: 1.10, 95% CI 1.00-1.22; (66) and Xuan D, et al. mentions both overweight and obesity as factors associated with stomach tumor. (67) On the other hand, Myon J. points to overweight/obesity as a protective factor.(56)

Hurtado S, et all, points out inadequate diet (low fruit and vegetable intake) as a risk factor associated with gastric neoplasia with a RR: 0.98 (0.73, 1.31) (68) and Umpiérrez I, et all. in their descriptive study, mention a low intake of fruits and vegetables in 36%, predominantly in women (69). In the present study the low consumption of fruits (x2 = 4.6599, p=0.0309) and vegetables (x2=7.2838, p=0.00070) was found to have a significant association with the presence of cancer. The results coincide with Ovidio Requejo and Hortensia García where they describe that the consumption of fruits and vegetables is a protective factor for gastric cancer. (70) Montes V, et al also conclude that a high consumption of fruits and vegetables decreases the risk of GC. (10)

The gender with the highest frequency of gastric cancer was male. This coincides with the study of Ortiz and Rodriguez i n which they indicate that 62% of this gender was affected (61). Similarly, in the study of Eulogio F. and Narciso R. the occurrence of the disease in the male gender was higher (71). Junfu Ma and Xin Hu also agree that gender is a critical factor in relation to gastric cancer (72). In a study developed in Peru, it is mentioned that the gender most affected in presenting gastric cancer was female. (73) In contrast, the study by Pantigoso L. indicates that gender is not a risk factor for developing gastric cancer. (74) For Helicobacter pylori infection, no significant association was found with gastric cancer (74).

gastric. This finding coincides with a Peruvian case-control study with an OR=0.28 (0.11-1.69) p=0.0023. (64) In contrast, studies developed by: Piazuelo et al; (75) León L. (76). Ushiku T. (77) and Hernando Marulanda, relate enterobacteria as a risk factor for the development of this neoplasia (78).

With respect to the variable family history, this variable was statistically significant, which coincides with that described by Castro M., in his research with an OR:6.729; 95%CI 4.049-11.184; (79) Chávez M. also refers that this variable is significant (80). On the other hand, socioeconomic level was statistically significant in our research, which coincides with Dianqin S. and Lin I. in their population-based study where it is concluded that socioeconomic level is a predisposing factor for gastric cancer with a RR 0.83 (0.74, 0.93) and a p=0.005.

CONCLUSIONS

1.   Premalignant lesions (gastric atrophy, metaplasia and dysplasia) were not found to be related to gastric cancer in patients of the gastroenterology service of hospital II Essalud Huánuco 2022.

2.   Overweight/obesity is not related to gastric cancer in patients of the gastroenterology service of hospital II Essalud Huánuco 2022.

3.   The low consumption of fruits and vegetables is related to gastric cancer in patients of the gastroenterology service of the hospital II Essalud Huánuco 2022, since a significant association was found with the consumption of fruits and vegetables.

BIBLIOGRAPHIC REFERENCES

1.   Valdivieso M. Gastric carcinoma: Risk factors. Role of Helicobacter pylori. DIAGN. 2021;60(2):7.

2.   Murillo B, Umaña B, Membreño M, Martínez B. Gastric carcinoma: literature review. Rev Med Leg COSTA H RICA. 2020;37(1):12.

3.   Sanchez DG, Moreira OD, Toste MA. Update on risk factors associated with gastric cancer mortality. Rev Habanera Cienc Médicas. 2021;20(5):8.

4.   On On Chan A, Wong B. Risk factors for gastric cancer - UpToDate [Internet]. UpToDate. 2022 [cited 2022 Nov 10]. Available from: https://www.uptodate.com/contents/risk-factors-for-gastric-cancer?search=Factors%20of%20risk%20of%20c%C3%A1ncer%20g%C3%Alstrico&source=search_result&selectedTitle=1~150&usage_type=default&displa y_rank=1.

5.   Cárdenas CE, Cárdenas JC, Játiva JJ. Câncer Gástrico: una revisão bibliográfica Gastric Cancer: a bibliographic review Câncer gástrico: uma revisão bibliográfica. 2021; 7:17.

6.   Shao L, Li P, Ye J, Chen J, Han Y, Cai J, et al. Risk of gastric cancer among patients with gastric intestinal metaplasia. International Journal of Cancer. 2018;143(7):1671-7.

7.   Friedenreich CM, Ryder C, McNeil J. Physical activity, obesity and sedentary behavior in cancer etiology: epidemiologic evidence and biologic mechanisms. Molecular Oncology. 2021;15(3):790-800.

8.   Ferro A, Costa AR, Morais S, Bertuccio P, Rota M, Pelucchi C, et al. Fruits and vegetables intake and gastric cancer risk: A pooled analysis within the Stomach cancer Pooling Project. International Journal of Cancer. 2020;147(11):3090-101.

9.   Poorolajal J, Moradi L, Mohammadi Y, Cheraghi Z, Gohari-Ensaf F. Risk factors for stomach cancer: a systematic review and meta-analysis. Epidemiol

Health. Feb 2, 2020; 42:8.

10.   Montes V, Rigotti E, Dathe S, Jara P, Brenner P, Gonzalez MT, Hofmann F. INTERNATIONAL STRATEGIES FOR THE PREVENTION OF GASTRIC CANCER. Confluencia Journal. 2021; 4(1): 78-83. Available at: https://revistas.udd.cl/index.php/confluencia/article/view/590/514

11.   Oliveros R, Pinilla R, Facundo H, Sanchez R. Gastric cancer: a preventable disease. Strategies for intervention in natural history. Rev Colomb Gastroenterol. 2019;34(2).

12.   Hurtado S, Trius M, Lamuela RM, Zamora R. Vegetable and Fruit Consumption and Prognosis Among Cancer Survivors: A Systematic Review and Meta-Analysis of Cohort Studies. Advances in Nutrition. Nov 15, 2020;11(6):1569-82.

13.   Palmero Picazo J, Tron Gómez MS, Tovar Torres S. Gastric cancer. Atención Familiar. Oct 10, 2018;25(4):169.

14.   Bedoya HA, Calvache C, Anduquia F, Hurtado N, Bedoya S, Ramirez C, et al. Premalignant and malignant lesions of the stomach in patients not screened for gastric cancer. Rev Colomb Cir. 2020; 35(04):570-4.

15.   Abadía J, Hernández J, Rodrigo A. Literature review of gastric cancer. Revista Brújula, Semilleros de Investigación. 2018;6(11):26-34.

16.   Ríos J. Stomach cancer: clinical presentation and general aspects. DIAGNOSIS. 2021;60(2):06.

17.   Buján S, Bolaños S, Mora K, Bolaños I. Gastric carcinoma: literature review. JOURNAL FORENSIC MEDICINE OF COSTA RICA. 2020;37(1):12.

18.   Gu L, Zhang Y, Hong J, Xu B, Yang L, Yan K, et al. Prognostic Value of Pretreatment Overweight/Obesity and Adipose Tissue Distribution in Resectable Gastric Cancer: A Retrospective Cohort Study. Frontiers in Oncology [Internet]. 2021 [cited May 24, 2022];11. Available from: https://www.frontiersin.org/article/10.3389/fonc.2021.680190

19.   Amiry F, Mousavi SM, Barekzai AM, Esmaillzadeh A. Adherence to the Mediterranean Diet in Relation to Gastric Cancer in Afghanistan. Frontiers in Nutrition [Internet]. 2022 [cited 2022 May 23, 2022];9. Available from: https://www.frontiersin.org/article/10.3389/fnut.2022.830646

20.   Mendoza C. Conditions associated with the development of gastric cancer in hospitalized patients of the gastroenterology service of the arzobispo loayza national hospital during 2018. [Lima]: Universidad privada San Juan Bautista; 2018.

21.   Castro M. Clinical-Epidemiological Factors Associated with Gastric Cancer in Patients Hospitalized in the Medical Services of the Dos de Mayo National Hospital, Period 2018 [licenciatura]. [Lima]: Universidad Privada San Juan Bautista; 2020.

22.   Paucar E. "Factors associated with the development of gastric cancer in patients at the adolfo guevara velasco national hospital in cusco, 2013-2018." [Cusco]: NATIONAL UNIVERSITY OF SAN ANTONIO ABAD DEL CUSCO; 2018.

23.   Quispe S. Dietary Patterns Associated with Gastric Cancer in Patients Attended at the Regional Institute of Neoplastic Diseases - North, July October 2014. [Trujillo]: Cesar Vallejo; 2014.

24.   Eulogio F, Narciso R. Factors related to Gastric Cancer in a Public Hospital of Huanuco. Rev Peru Investig Salud. 2018;2(1):42-49.

25.   Rodríguez P. Sociodemographic factors (education level, geographical location), harmful habits (tobacco and alcohol), eating habits (salt, smoked meat, reheated food) and food preservation (use of refrigerator and insecticides); associated with gastric cancer with endoscopic diagnosis, in patients of the gastroenterology service of the regional hospital Hermilio Valdizán, from 2015 to 2017, Huánuco - Peru [licenciatura]. [Huánuco]: Hermilio Valdizan Medrano; 2019.

26.Vincent T. Cancer Principles & Practice of Oncology. In: Cancer Principles & Practice of Oncology. 11th ed. London; 2015. p. 400-50.

27.   Galindo F, Daneri G. Gastric carcinoma. In: Galindo F, et al, editors. Encyclopedia Digestive Surgery. 2020. p. 1-67. (223; vol. volume II).

28.   Avital I, Nissan A, Golan T, Lawrence YR, Stojadinovic A. Cancer of the Stomach. In: DeVita V, Lawrence T, Rosenberg S, editors. Cancer Principles & Practice of Oncology. 11th ed. Copyright 2019 Wolters Kluwer; 2019. p. 1386-446.

29.   Medrano R, García L, Luna M. Gastric cancer. In: Rivera Rivera S, editor. GENERAL ONCOLOGY FOR HEALTH CARE PROFESSIONALS OF THE FIRST CONTACT. Mexico: Permanyer México; 2017. p. 127-34.

30.   Rojas V, Montagné N. Overview of gastric cancer. RC_UCR-HSJD [Internet]. April 30, 2019 [cited June 20, 2022];9(2). Available from: https://revistas.ucr.ac.cr/index.php/clinica/article/view/37351

31.   Rollán A, Cortés P, Calvo A, Araya R, Bufadel ME, González R, et al. Early diagnosis of gastric cancer: proposal for detection and follow-up of gastric premalignant lesions: ACHED protocol. Rev méd Chile. 2014;142(9):1181-92.

32.   Csendes A, Figueroa M. Status of gastric cancer in the world and in Chile. Revista Chilena de Cirugía. 2017;69(6):502-7.

33.   Ruiz D, Téllez FI, Barreto R, Zamora LE. Prevention, screening and endoscopic follow-up of premalignant lesions of the upper and middle digestive tract. Endoscopy. 2015;27(3):135-45.

34.   Grajales G, Téllez FI, Barreto R. Scrutiny and follow-up of premalignant lesions of the upper gastrointestinal tract. Endoscopy 2013; 25(3): 123-132.

35.   Romero J, Bello M. Digestive cancer seen from dynamics: flat lesions of the gastrointestinal mucosa and dysplasia. April 16 Journal. 2018;57(268):135-44.

36.   Juantá J, Sancho D, Loría L, Rojas F. GASTRIC DYSPLASIA, EXPERIENCE. AT THE SAN JUAN DE DIOS HOSPITAL 2004-2008. Clinical Journal of the UCR School of Medicine - HSJD. 2012;2(X):7.

37.   Moreno M. Definición y clasificación de la obesidad /Definition and classification of obesity. Rev. Méd. Clín. Condes. 2012;23(2):124-128.

38.   Perreault L. Obesity in adults: Etiologies and risk factors [Internet]. UptoDate. 2022 [cited 2022 Jun 10, 2022]. Available from: https://www.uptodate.com/contents/obesity-in-adults-etiologies-and-risk-factors?search=obesity&source=search_result&selectedTitle=9~150&usage_type =d efault&display_rank=9

39.   Zhang S, Wang JB, Yang H, Fan JH, Qiao YL, Taylor PR. Body mass index and risk of upper gastrointestinal cancer: A 30-year follow-up of the Linxian dysplasia nutrition intervention trial cohort. Cancer Epidemiology. 2020; 65:101683.

40.   Aoyama T, Nakazono M, Nagasawa S, Segami K. Clinical Impact of a Perioperative Exercise Program for Sarcopenia and Overweight/Obesity Gastric Cancer. In Vivo. 2021;35(2):707-12

41.   Skelton JW. Definition, epidemiology, and etiology of obesity in children and adolescents. October 8, 2021 [cited 2021 June 10, 2022]; Available from: https://www.uptodate.com/contents/definition-epidemiology-and-etiology-of-obesity-in-children-and

42.   Suárez W, Sánchez AJ, González JA, Suárez W, Sánchez AJ, González JA. Pathophysiology of obesity: current perspective. Chilean journal of nutrition. 2017;44(3):226-33.

43.   Suarez W, Sanchez A. Body mass index: advantages and disadvantages of its use nobesity. Relationship with strength and physical activity. Nov 28, 2018; 7:128-39.

44.   Aráuz JDD. Obesity: Pathophysiology and Management Strategies. 2021;

49. 45.Laviada H, Molina Segui F. Pathophysiology of obesity and weight defense.
body. In: Pathophysiology of obesity [Internet]. 2021. Available from:

https://www.researchgate.net/publication/356391301

46. Metere A, Giacomelli L. Absorption, metabolism and protective role of fruits and vegetables polyphenols against gastric cancer. :9.

47. Graham Colditz, Classification of fruits and vegetables . Healthy diet in adults. [Internet]. UptoDate. 2019 [cited June 14, 2022]. Available from: https://www.uptodate.com/contents/healthy-diet-in

48. FAO. Fruits and vegetables - essential in your diet [Internet]. 2020 [cited June 14, 2022]. Available from:

49. http://www.fao.org/documents/card/en/c/cb2395es

50. Rodriguez M. Challenges to fruit and vegetable consumption. Journal of the Faculty of Human Medicine. April 2019;19(2):105-12.

51. Ferro A, Costa AR, Morais S, Bertuccio P, Rota M, Pelucchi C, et al. Fruits and vegetables intake and gastric cancer risk: A pooled analysis within the Stomach cancer Pooling Project. International Journal of Cancer. 2020;147(11):3090-101.

52. Hurtado-Barroso S, Trius-Soler M, Lamuela-Raventós RM, Zamora-Ros R. Vegetable and Fruit Consumption and Prognosis Among Cancer Survivors: A Systematic Review and Meta-Analysis of Cohort Studies. Advances in Nutrition. Nov 15, 2020;11(6):1569-82.

53. García Rodríguez M, Romero Saldaña M, Alcaide Leyva JM, Moreno Rojas R, Molina Recio G. Design and validation of a food frequency questionnaire (FFQ) for the nutritional evaluation of food intake in the Peruvian Amazon. J Health Popul Nutr. December 2019;38(1):47.

54. Bertuccio P, Rosato V, Andreano A, Ferraroni M, Decarli A, Edefonti V, et al. Dietary patterns and gastric cancer risk: a systematic review and meta-analysis. Annals of Oncology. 2013 June;24(6):1450-8.

55. Steevens J, Schouten LJ, Goldbohm RA, van den Brandt PA. Vegetables and fruits consumption and risk of esophageal and gastric cancer subtypes in the

Netherlands Cohort Study. International Journal of Cancer. 2011;129(11):2681-93.

56. Barajas JCL. Physiopathology and nutrition. Page Six; 2021. 225 p.

57. Myon J. Body Mass Index and Risk of Gastric Cancer in Asian Adults: A Meta- Epidemiological Meta-Analysis of Population-Based Cohort Studies. Cancer Res Treat. 2020;52(2):369-373. https://doi.org/10.4143/crt.2019.241.

58. Martínez D, Arzeta V, Jiménez H, Román A, Fernández G. Stomach cancer: risk factors, diagnosis and treatment. AyTBUAP. 2021; 6(23):52-71.

59. Ministry of Health of Peru/ National Center for Epidemiology, Prevention and Disease Control. Analysis of the situation of Cancer in Peru, 2018.

60. Akbari M, Tabrizi R, Kardeh S, Lankarani K. Gastric cancer in patients with gastric atrophy and intestinal metaplasia: A systematic review and meta-analysis. PLOS ONE. 2019;14(7)

61. Spence A, Cardwell C, McMenamin U, Hicks B, Johnston B. Adenocarcinoma risk in gastric atrophy and intestinal metaplasia: a systematic review. 2017; 17 (57).

62. Ortiz J, Rodríguez S, Olarte G. Sociodemographic, environmental and clinical characteristics. in patients with gastric cancer in San Gil, Colombia. Rev Enferm Inst Mex Seguro Soc. 2021; 29 (3): 136-141.

63. Jonathan WJ, Lee feng zhu. Severity of gastric intestinal metaplasia predicts gastric cancer risk: a multicenter prospective cohort study (GCEP). 2022 May;71(5):854-863.

64. Rollán A, et al. Recommendations of the Chilean association for digestive endoscopy for the management of gastric pre-malignant lesions. Rev. med. chile. 2014; 142(9).

65. Paucar E. Factors associated with the development of gastric cancer in patients of the Adolfo Guevara Velasco national hospital of Cusco, 2013-2018 [licenciatura]. [Pucallpa]: National University of San Antonio Abad del Cusco;

2019.

66.   Vallejo Parada D, Orellana Tapia M, Trepat Vidal G. Gastric cancer and bariatric surgery: a case report. Rev. Cirugia. 2022;74(6). Available at: doi:10.35687/s2452-454920220061585 [Accessed 12 Jan. 2023].

67.   Jun X, Peng C, Dong X, Kang Y, Shuang L, Hong H, Yu L, Liu X. Body Mass Index and Risk of Gastric Cancer: A Meta-analysis. Jpn J Clin Oncol. 2014; 44(9):783- 791.

68.   Xuan D, Hidayat K, Min B. Abdominal obesity and gastroesophageal cancer risk: systematic review and meta-analysis of prospective studies. Biosciencie Reports. 2017; 37.

69.   Hurtado S, Trius M, Lamuela R, Zamora R. Vegetable and Fruit Consumption and Prognosis Among Cancer Survivors: A Systematic Review and Meta-Analysis of Cohort Studies. Adv Nutr. 2020; 11:1569-1582. https://doi.org/10.1093/advances/nmaa082.

70.   Umpiérrez I, Martin JC, Rodríguez L, Cambet Y, García B. Clinical, endoscopic and histologic behavior of gastric cancer diagnosed at the "Dr. Mario Muñoz Monroy" Hospital. Rev Med Electron. 2020; 42 (6).

71.   Ovid H, Garcia H. Mediterranean diet and cancer. Nutrition Hosp. 2021; 38(2): 71- 74.

72.   Eulogio F, Narciso R. Factors related to Gastric Cancer in a Public Hospital of Huanuco. Rev Peru Investig Salud. 2018;2(1):42-49.

73.   Junfu Ma 1, Xin Hu. Characterization of two ferroptosis subtypes with distinct immune infiltration and gender difference in gastric cancer. 2021; 8: 756193.

74.   Carrillo, S. and Delzo, J. Epidemiological characteristics of patients with gastric cancer at the Regional Institute of Neoplastic Diseases of the Center, Junín 2020-2021 [undergraduate]. [Huancayo]: Universidad Continental, Huancayo; 2022.

75.   Pantigoso L. Risk factors associated with gastric cancer in patients attended at the amazon hospital during the period 2016 to 2017 [licenciatura]. [Pucallpa]: National University of Ucayali; 2021.

76.   Piazuelo B, Bravo L, Mera R, Constanza M, Bravo J, Delgado A, et al. The Colombian Chemoprevention Trial: 20-Year Follow-Up of a Cohort of Patients With Gastric Precancerous Lesions. Gastroenterology. 2021; 160 (4): 1106 - 1117.

77.   León L. Evaluation of the dietary pattern in patients with screening and diagnosis of gastric cancer associated with Helicobacter pylori at the National Institute of Neoplastic Diseases [licenciatura]. [Lima]: Universidad Nacional Mayor de San Marcos; 2020.

78.   Ushiku T, Abe H. - Pathologic diversity of gastric cancer from the viewpoint of background condition. 2022; 103(1).

79.   Marulanda H, Otero W, Gomez M. Helicobacter pylori, nodular gastritis and premalignant lesions of the stomach: a case-control study. Rev. gastroenterol. 2018; 38(4).

80.   Castro M. Clinical - Epidemiological Factors Associated with Gastric Cancer in Patients Hospitalized in the Medical Services of the Dos de Mayo National Hospital, Period 2018 [licenciatura]. [Lima]: Universidad Privada San Juan Bautista; 2020.

81.   Chávez M, Tanimoto M - Mexican consensus on the detection and treatment of early gastric cancer. The Mexican consensus on the detection and treatment of early gastric cancer. Rev. de Gastroenterología de México. 2020; 85(1): 69-85.

82.   Sol Dianqin, lin lei - Sociodemographic disparities in gastric cancer and gastric precancerous cascade: a population-based study. VOLUME 23, 100437 ,01 JUNE 2022.

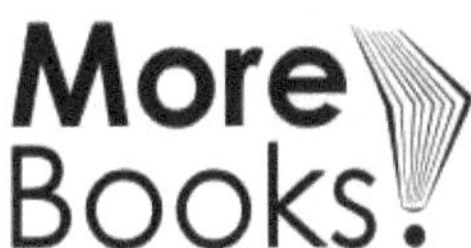
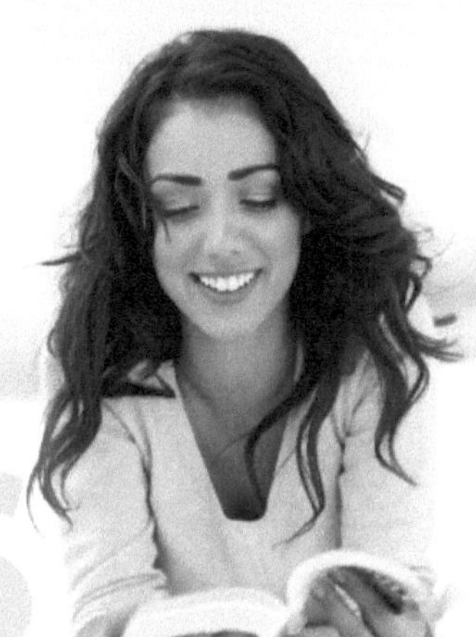

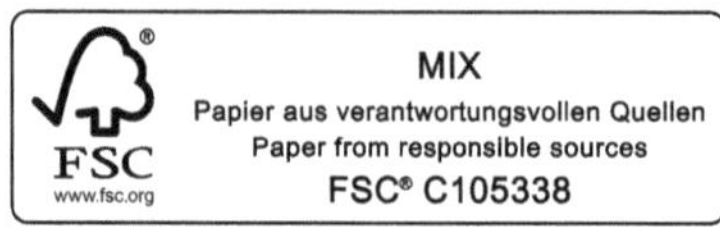

Printed by Books on Demand GmbH, Norderstedt / Germany